F_{abulous} A_{nd} T_{riumphant}

Lose Weight Without Losing Your Mind

Bethany Calvo Buides

March 2017

To my husband Nibaldo: and my children Shelby and Dimitri. You inspire me every day to be the best person I can be. Thank you for loving and supporting me and to God for helping me get through the challenging days. Anything is possible if you just believe.

Disclaimer

Please consult your physician before starting this or any other fitness and meal plan. This plan worked for me and I hope it works for you, however, do not take a risk without checking with your physician first. Always remember that your health and well-being come first.

Introduction

For most of my life I have been overweight and for most of that time it really didn't bother me. I was raised to be super confident in who I am and what I have to offer the world, so I felt very comfortable in my own skin. Sure there were a few times when I said to myself "Ugh, I got to do something about this weight." But for the most part I just went on eating and living my life like everything was okay. When I started my weight loss journey this time I didn't even give it much thought and I didn't have a plan at first and maybe that was the key to being so successful. Many people have come up to me and asked how I lost 75 pounds in just 7 months, so my husband suggested I write this book about my journey. As you read through the pages, I hope you find inspiration and some ideas to help you become more fit in your life.

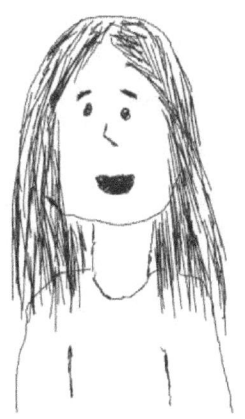

Are you ready to change your life?

Content

Get Up and Move!!!!!

Seriously get up right now and move!!!! I know you are trying to read this book but you need to get up and move for at least five minutes. Shake it, twist it, twerk it, I don't care how you do it just move. Don't worry I will be here when you get back. Phew!!! Now we have your blood pumping. Just admit it, you feel really good right? Guess what? You just made your first move to a healthier you. I am super proud of you!!!!!

I remember how I started my journey. I was outside at work on lunch and I was sitting down at a picnic table. It was a beautiful day and it felt great to get out of the building. I should mention that I work in an office where a majority of my day is sitting at a computer. I was 46 years old and 314 pounds with bad knees and spent most of my days sedentary. As I was sitting there I thought to myself that I should stand up and walk around the building one time and see how it feels. So I did and it wasn't bad. I felt a little out of breath and my body hurt but I did it. So I walked around another time and then another. At that point I was completely out of breath and my body still hurt but I felt pretty good about my accomplishment.

The next day I tried walking around the building four times and I did it and I was super excited. As weeks passed I found myself progressing more and more with my speed and duration. What was even cooler is that my co-workers and strangers were coming up to me telling me that they noticed me walking and they were so impressed and that I was motivating them to start moving. When I realized that people were watching I felt more inclined to want to push myself more and more. I thought to myself if I can just motivate one person to move I need to do it. Even on days when I felt like I didn't want to walk I pushed myself to do it just in case someone was watching and needed motivation. It must be said, that I wasn't losing weight and getting fit for others. I was moving and getting fit for myself, but I have to say it was a great motivator knowing that maybe I could inspire someone out there just by moving myself.

Now that I started moving more and feeling more motivated I thought that I might try to do something about what I was eating. At this point I had only been moving and I lost about 5 or so pounds in just a couple of weeks. Who knows how much I would lose if I actually changed what I was eating?

It's <u>Not</u> All Fun and Games

Let's talk about eating shall we? I love love love to eat, especially nachos, chili hot dogs and pizza. Who is with me? I think for most folks it is hard to know which diet program to choose from. I had tried so many in the past and failed at each and every one. Sometimes I quit because I was hungry all the time and other times I stopped trying because I couldn't eat what I wanted. There was always something that made me go back to my bad eating habits.

After researching online I decided to go with a low carb/high protein diet. It seemed like the best choice for what I needed to be able to stick to the plan. It was important for me to choose something that I could follow indefinitely. I basically consumed no more than 20 grams of carbohydrates a day. I didn't have to watch calories or fat. I ate as much as I wanted as long as I stayed below the 20 grams of carbs. The great thing about low carbs and high protein is you never go hungry. Sure there were cravings but I definitely felt full after eating. Don't worry, later in the book I will break down each phase that I went through to lose the weight.

So my goal was to consume 20 grams of carbs or less a day for two weeks. I didn't want to do it for longer than a couple of weeks because I didn't know if I would stick to it. I stayed on this plan for around two weeks and lost 15 pounds!!!! Yep I know that is pretty amazing right? There were a few days when I just wanted a french fry so bad that I would fantasize about it throughout the day.

I can't say that those two weeks were easy because they were not. Again, I didn't feel hungry at all but I just wanted more carbs and I couldn't have them. There were a lot of cravings and believe me I had to do a lot of praying during this time asking for the will power to get through. The plus side to this program is that I was able to eat as much meat and other proteins as I wanted as long as it didn't have carbs. This means I had all the bacon, chicken, fish, hamburger and pork that I wanted. Don't worry Vegetarians and Vegans, there are plenty of protein alternatives to meat so as long as you are consuming a considerable amount of protein and keeping your carbs at 20 grams you will do well on this program as well. I had to get a little creative when it came to low carb recipes but I found a way to make it work and began embracing the whole low carb lifestyle.

After the two weeks were over I started adding more and more carbs to my diet but rarely exceeded 50 grams a day. I prefer to stay under 50 grams of carbs most days but if I want to splurge a little I go up to 100 grams. I completely cut out bread and pasta. This was rather easy for me because I never craved these before the program.

I look at each and every label to see how many carbs are in that item. If I don't have the label I look online so that I can get a general I idea. You would be surprised the amounts of carbs in some foods, especially in sugar free foods and "diet" foods. Some of these foods have more carbs than eating something with real sugar in it. For example, the amount of carbs in a regular cup of vanilla ice cream is less than the carbs in a sugar free cup of vanilla ice cream depending on the brand. Isn't that crazy??

The most important thing is choosing the right food. There are days that I splurge and have something that I really want and on these days I choose the lesser of the two evils. If you are really craving pizza, eat pizza but get thin crust or even better eat it without the crust. If you are craving a doughnut eat a cookie instead. Look at the carbs and pick the one with less carbs. You will feel satisfied but you will not be consuming so many carbs. It is all about choosing better. I have not eaten a hamburger bun in about 8 months, but I have eaten a heck of a lot of hamburgers. This has become a way of life for me now and I don't really feel like I am depriving myself of anything. I feel completely sated.

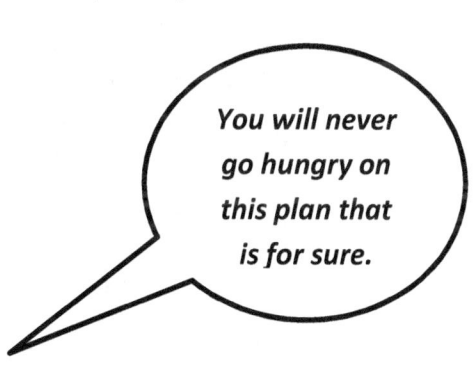

You will never go hungry on this plan that is for sure.

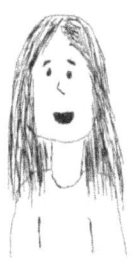

Stepping and Dancing in the Stall

In the first chapter I spoke about walking and how I made sure that I was moving often. Around 4 months into my weight loss program I decided to purchase a step tracker. There are so many to choose from and if you want to save money you can download a free step tracker on your cell phone. I recommend a step tracker that you wear on your wrist or around your neck. These trackers seem to be more accurate. The step tracker brought my fitness up to another level. We are told that 10,000 steps a day should be the bare minimum goal for most people. So for the first week I made sure I that I achieved that goal. I made most of my steps by dancing in my living room in front of the TV watching one of my favorite shows or a movie. I liked the distraction and before I knew it was completing 15,000 steps a day and then 20,000 and then

25,000. I found the need to complete the steps a bit addicting. I wanted to challenge myself to move more. My husband and I would compete with each other to see how many steps we could do in one day. It's fun when you can have someone to challenge you.

Let's talk about dancing in restroom stalls. Yep, you read that right I said restroom stalls. I make sure I keep moving and get my steps in no matter the location even if that means dancing in restrooms. Remember when I said that I work in an office and that my work is very sedentary? Well I have to do something to offset all of that sitting, so I get up every hour and walk over to the restroom and dance in one of the stalls for a couple of minutes. Sure this isn't the ideal way of getting my steps in but oh does it work, especially on rainy or cold days when I cannot exercise outside. There are some days when I dance in the stall during all three of my breaks. At first I was a little hesitant, because I was worried about what people might think, hearing me stomp around, but then I thought to myself "I am losing weight so who cares what people think". I typically complete around 8,000 to 10,000 steps before I leave work for the day, so it really does make a difference. What's so funny is that I told some of my co-workers about it and now some of them are working out in the restroom stall too. Before you know it, we will have to take reservations for the dance party in the restroom!!! Whether it is dancing in the restrooms or walking or biking. The goal is to move every chance you get.

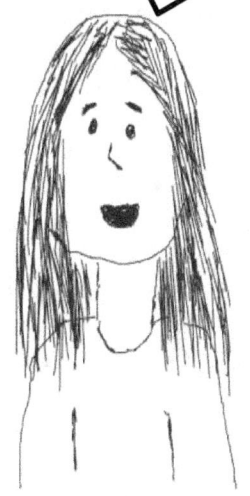

Accepting Yourself Now and Forever

We have talked about moving and eating right; let's talk a little about acceptance. We all have different reasons for wanting to lose weight and becoming fit, just make sure that the reason is you. I say this because in the past I let society dictate to me what the ideal size should be and I let society make me feel bad when I felt like I couldn't live up to the people in the magazine's and on television. We live in a world where technology affects us in more ways than it has ever before. Whether it be social media, movies, videos or other mediums we are made to believe that if you are not "skinny" you do not matter. Don't let this get to you. Drown out all of the negative energy and don't be afraid to dance to the beat of your own drum. Look at yourself in the mirror and say "I am beautiful, I am strong, I am fierce and I am worthy." It is so important to accept yourself just the way you are. You should be motivated to lose weight so that you can feel better and become a healthier you. There will be days when you slip up and eat something you shouldn't eat or you don't move as much as you should but that is okay because you can try again the next day and the next and the next until you get to where you want to be. You are in the driver's seat and you control what you eat and how you move and I know without a shadow of a doubt that you will do this!!! You will become a better you and feel wonderful about what you have accomplished. If I can do it, anyone can, all you have to do is make the first move.

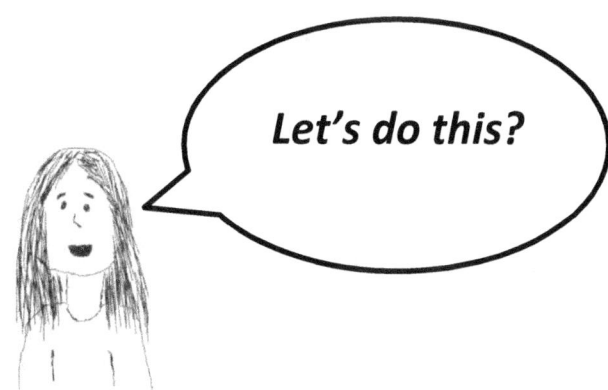

The Plan

Phase 1

Weeks 1 and 2

During the first two weeks you will consume 20 grams of carbs or less and complete 15,000 steps per day. Try your very best to not go over 20 grams, otherwise you may not see such a dramatic loss of weight. Remember that you choose your carbs so there isn't really a rule about what kind of carbs you consume, however I highly suggest that you use a big portion of your carbs for vegetables every day. I have never been a big fan of vegetables so I was a bit limited with my choices. However, I made sure that I had vegetables every day to ensure that I consumed plenty of vitamins and fiber. Vegetables high in fiber will help you feel full faster and of course consuming a lot of lean protein will have the same effect. You shouldn't feel hungry during these two weeks because you are eating as much as you want of carb free proteins. If you feel a craving for something sweet I suggest sugar free chewing gum or sugar free mints. Please keep in mind that these typically have 1 to 2 grams of carbs and should be monitored so that you don't carb out on gum or mints. I would sometimes drink a sugar free beverage when I was craving something sweet, it helped me with cravings as well.

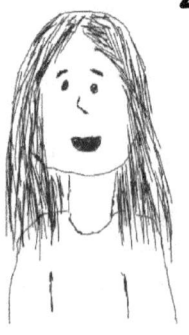

Don't eat that doughnut!!!! It is not worth it. Keep focused on your goal.

Phase 2

Weeks 3 and 4

You did it!!!! You made it through the first two weeks of what I like to call the longest two weeks ever!!!! ☺ By now you should have noticed some weight loss and an increased energy level. I am super proud of your progress. How about we add some more carbs to your daily intake? Sounds good right??? Let's bump up your carb intake to 30 grams of carbs and your steps to 20,000 per day. An additional 10 grams of carbs may not seem like a lot but you would be surprised what a difference it makes. You can add more fruit if you like and maybe even a low carb ice cream, but don't go crazy with it, just a little okay? You should feel so much better during weeks 3 and 4 because you are consuming more carbs and moving more. There should be a lot more dancing to make sure you complete those 20,000 steps or whatever exercise you prefer just make sure you get those steps in so that you can continue to lose weight and become healthier.

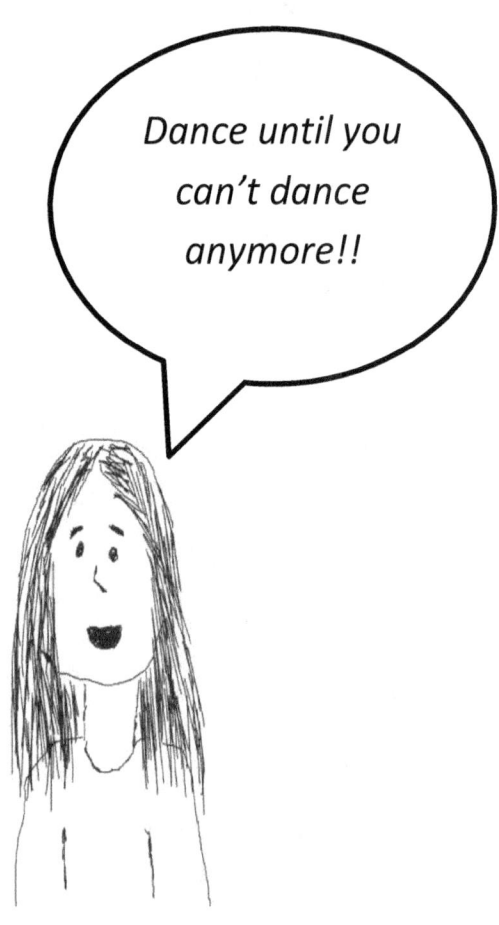

Dance until you can't dance anymore!!

Phase 3

Months 2, 3, 4 and 5

If you have made it to this page you have successfully completed a whole month of this program. Woohoo!!!! I knew you could do it!!! Now we can move up your carbs to 50 grams per day and 25,000 steps. I know that 25,000 may seem like a lot but we need to make up for the extra carbs you are consuming. Its only 5,000 more than last week and you know you can do it. So get to stepping already!! By now you have learned a lot about carbs and which ones are better than others, so it should be very easy to add 20 more grams of carbs to your daily intake. As long as you follow this plan you will continue to lose weight and get fit.

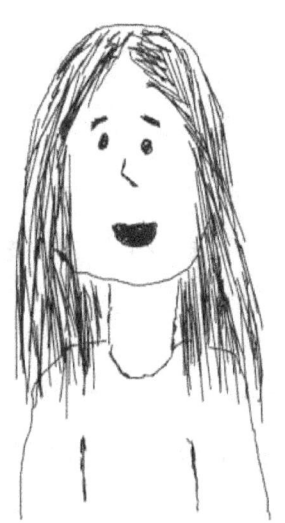

Phase 4

Maintenance

Wow, you have now finished 5 months and I am pretty sure that you are happy about your progress right? I mean who would have thought that these past 5 months would fly by and you would lose so much weight and feel so great. I don't even recognize you anymore and that's a good thing. If at this time you have lost all of the weight that you wanted to lose then I say bump up your carb consumption to 75 grams and make sure that you continue to complete 25,000 steps a day. Check your weight every week to make sure that you are maintaining your weight and adjust the carb intake if you see that you are gaining again. If you haven't lost all the weight that you want that's okay, just maintain the 50 grams of carbs and 25,000 steps until you get to your ideal weight or size. Even now after 7 months I still keep my carb consumption to 50 grams of carbs a day because I want to lose a little more weight. I have days when I splurge a bit and that is okay, because we all need that every once and while. Just make sure you get right back to the plan the very next day. Every person's body and metabolism is different so it may take you longer to lose the weight but don't worry you will get there. If you find that you want to splurge one day and eat more carbs you can do that, just don't falter on your steps. I can't tell you how important it is to make sure you are completing at least 25,000 steps a day. At this point on the plan anything less might make you gain some weight back and we don't want that. Keep track of carbs and steps and see what works for you once you have lost all of your weight. There is a magic number for everyone and you will find yours with a little practice.

Eventually you will not have to count carbs because you will know how many carbs are in the foods you eat and you will know how much you can consume. Keep in mind that this is a way of life for you now. It is not a diet, it is a live it! You have to hold yourself accountable for what you eat and how often you move. There will come a time when this program will become effortless for you and you won't remember living any other way.

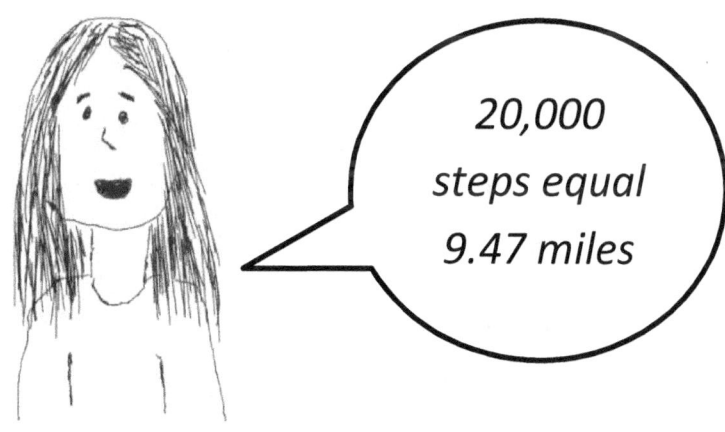

Low Carb Vegetables

Arugula: One, cup of arugula contains 1 gram of carbs.

Asparagus: One, half-cup of cooked asparagus contains 3.5 grams of carbs.

Broccoli: One, cup of broccoli contains 6 grams of carbs

Cauliflower: One, cup of cooked cauliflower contains 5 grams of carbs.

Celery: Two medium stalks of celery contain 2.5 grams of carbs.

Cucumber: One, half-cup of sliced cucumber contains 2 grams of carbs.

Green Leaf lettuce: One, cup of green leaf lettuce contains 1 gram of carbs.

Green Beans: One, cup of green beans contains 8 grams of carbs.

Green pepper: One, half-cup of sliced green peppers contains 2 grams of carbs.

Iceberg lettuce: One, cup of shredded iceberg lettuce contains 2 grams of carbs.

Kale: One, half-cup of chopped cooked kale contains 4 grams of carbs.

Okra: One, half-cup of cooked sliced okra contains 3.5 grams of carbs.

Radishes: One, half-cup of sliced raw radishes contains 2 grams of carbs.

Red bell pepper: One, half-cup of red pepper contains 3 grams of carbs.

Romaine lettuce: One cup of shredded romaine lettuce contains 1.5 grams of carbs

Spinach: One, half-cup of cooked spinach contains 3.5 grams of carbs.

Sugar snap peas: One, half-cup of whole raw sugar snap peas contains 1 gram of carbs.

Turnips: One, half- cup of cooked turnips contains 4 grams of carbs.

White mushrooms: One, half-cup of raw sliced white mushrooms contains 2 grams of carbs.

Yellow pepper: One, half-cup of sliced yellow pepper contains 3 grams of carbs.

Low Carb Fruits

Avocado: One, half-cup of an avocado contains 6.5 grams of carbs.

Blackberries: One, half-cup of blackberries contains 7 grams of carbs.

Blueberries: One, half-cup of blueberries contains 11 grams of carbs.

Cantaloupe: One, half-cup of cantaloupe contains 6.5 grams of carbs.

Cherries: One, half-cup of cherries contains 11 grams of carbs.

Clementine: One medium clementine contains 9 grams of carbs.

Cranberries: One half-cup of cranberries contains 6.5 grams of carbs.

Grapefruit: One half medium grapefruit contains 10.5 grams of carbs.

Honeydew Melon: One half-cup honeydew melon contains 8 grams of carbs.

Kiwi: One medium kiwi contains 11 grams of carbs.

Mango: One, half-cup of mango contains 14 grams of carbs.

Nectarines: One medium nectarine contains 15 grams of carbs.

Orange: One medium orange contains 15.5 grams of carbs.

Peaches: One medium peach contains 14.5 grams of carbs.

Pineapple: One, half-cup of pineapple chunks contains 11 grams of carbs.

Plums: One medium plum contains 7.5 grams of carbs.

Raspberries: One, half-cup of raspberries contains 7.5 grams of carbs.

Strawberries: One, half-cup of strawberries contains 5.5 grams of carbs.

Tangerines: One medium tangerine contains 12 grams of carbs.

Watermelon: One, half-cup of watermelon contains 5.5 grams of carbs.

Example Menu 1

Breakfast

3 pieces of bacon (0 carbs)

2 eggs (0 carbs)

1 slice of cheese (0 carbs)

Snack

14 almonds (2.5 carbs)

Lunch

1 cup of canned chicken (0 carbs)

2 cups of green leaf lettuce (2 carbs)

½ cup shredded cheese (0 carbs)

Snack

14 almonds (2.5 carbs)

Dinner

Un-Nacho (6)

½ cup of strawberries (5.5 carbs)

Total Carbs for the day 18.5

Example Menu 2

Breakfast

1 cup of smoked sausage (2 carbs)

2 eggs (0 carbs)

1 slice of cheese (0 carbs)

Snack

14 almonds (2.5 carbs)

Lunch

1 cup of ground beef (0 carbs)

2 cups of green leaf lettuce (2 carbs)

½ cup shredded cheese (0 carbs)

Snack

14 almonds (2.5 carbs)

Dinner

1 8 ounce chicken (0 carbs)

1 slice of cheese (0 carbs)

1 cup of cooked cauliflower (5 carbs)

½ cup of watermelon (5.5 carbs)

Total Carbs for the day 19.5

Example Menu 3

Breakfast

3 eggs (0 carbs)

¼ cup of shredded cheese (0 carbs)

Snack

14 almonds (2.5 carbs)

Lunch

12 ounce pork chop (0 carbs)

1 cup of broccoli (6 carbs)

1 slice of cheese (0 carbs)

Snack

14 almonds (2.5 carbs)

 Dinner

1 cup of cooked chicken (0 carbs)

1 slice of cheese (0 carbs)

2 cups of green leaf lettuce (2carbs)

½ cup of blackberries (7 carbs)

Total Carbs for the day 20

Broccoli and Cauliflower Casserole (6 grams of carbs per serving)

3 cups chopped Broccoli

3 cups chopped Cauliflower

½ cup 1% milk

1 cup shredded cheddar cheese

2 tsp. Onion Powder

2 tsp. Parmesan cheese

1 tsp. Salt

Directions: Heat oven to 350 degrees. Combine all ingredients except parmesan cheese in a 9X11 pan. Sprinkle parmesan cheese on top of mixture. Bake for 30 minutes. Feel free to add more seasoning if needed. Remember to always look at the nutritional information on the back of the seasoning because some seasonings contain carbs.

Chicken Goulash (6 grams of carbs per serving)

1 pound chicken breast

1 can petite tomatoes

2 Tbsp. cream cheese

2 tsp. Onion Powder

2 tsp. Garlic Powder

2 tsp. Parmesan cheese

1 tsp. Salt

Directions: Combine all ingredients in a skillet except for the tomatoes, cream cheese and parmesan. Cook until meat is done and add tomatoes, cream cheese and parmesan cover for 10 minutes. Feel free to add more seasoning if needed. Remember to always look at the nutritional information on the back of the seasoning because some seasonings contain carbs.

Hamburger Delight (6 grams carbs per serving)

1 pound lean ground beef

1 can petite tomatoes

2 Tbsp. cream cheese

2 tsp. Onion Powder

2 tsp. Garlic Powder

1 tsp. Salt

Directions: Combine all ingredients in a skillet except for the cream cheese and tomatoes. Cook until meat is done and add tomatoes and cream cheese and cover for 10 minutes. Feel free to add more seasoning if needed. Remember to always look at the nutritional information on the back of the seasoning because some seasonings contain carbs.

Bacon Wrap (5 grams of carbs per serving)

6 pieces bacon

2 large pieces of leaf lettuce

½ cup shredded cheddar cheese

1 tsp sour cream

Directions: Cook bacon thoroughly. Place bacon in the leaf lettuce and add cheese. The lettuce is a great substitute for a tortilla shell. Feel free to add more ingredients however, this may change carb consumption. If you do not like bacon you can choose another meat.

Un-Nachos (6 grams of carbs per serving)

1 pound ground beef

2 cups chopped green leaf lettuce

1 packet of taco seasoning

½ cup shredded cheddar cheese

2 tsp. Onion Powder

2 tsp. Garlic Powder

1 tsp. Salt

1 Tbsp. sour cream

Directions: Combine all ingredients in a skillet except for lettuce, cheese and sour cream Cook until meat is done. Place chopped lettuce on a plate and then add beef, cheddar cheese and sour cream. This can be for an individual meal or if you want to share. The crunchiness of the lettuce is a great substitute for tortilla chips. Feel free to add more seasoning if needed. Remember to always look at the nutritional information on the back of the seasoning because some seasonings contain carbs.

Un-Pizza (6 grams of carbs per serving)

1 pound ground beef

1 can tomato sauce

1 ounce of pepperoni

½ cup shredded mozzarella cheese

2 tsp. Onion Powder

2 tsp. Garlic Powder

1 tsp. Oregano

2 tsp. Parmesan cheese

1 tsp. Salt

Directions: Combine all ingredients in a skillet except for the mozzarella, pepperoni and parmesan. Cook until meat is done and add mozzarella, pepperoni and parmesan cover for 10 minutes. Feel free to add more seasoning if needed. Remember to always look at the nutritional information on the back of the seasoning because some seasonings contain carbs.

Things to Remember

- Set small and achievable goals

- Drink plenty of water

- Eat less and move more

- Allow yourself a splurge every once and awhile

- Challenge a friend to a step competition

- Eat more vegetables

- Get enough sleep

- Dance in a restroom stall

- Try new things

- Encourage others to move

And

Always Believe in Yourself!!!!!!!!

For before and after photos and

updates please visit:

www. fabulousandtriumphant.com

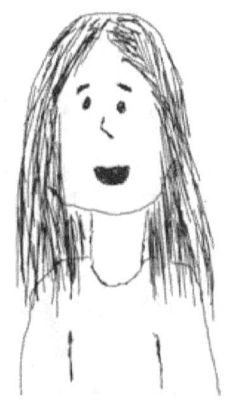

www.ingramcontent.com/pod-product-compliance
Lightning Source LLC
Chambersburg PA
CBHW071300280526
45788CB00004B/1783